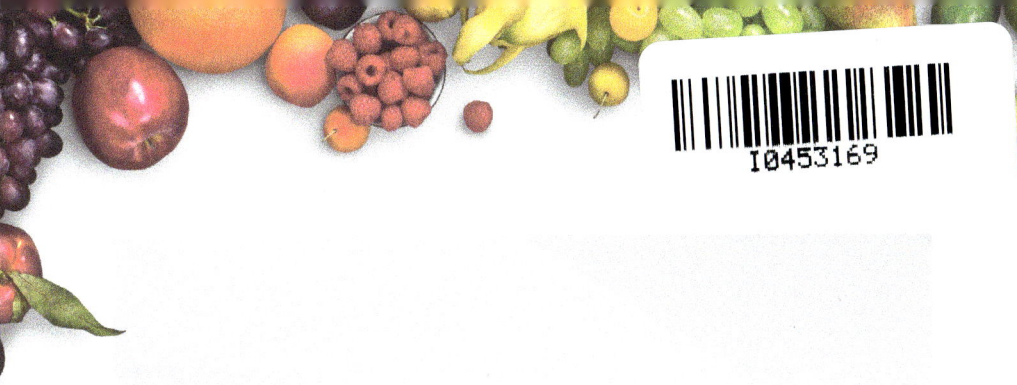

My name is Dr. Nora Shariff-Borden, I am the Founder of
The Kingdom Body Renewal Health & Wellness
Ministry is a faith-based initiative dedicated to helping
God's people renew their minds and transform the way
they think about food, health, and lifestyle. This ministry
is grounded in the belief that true wellness begins with a
renewed mind and a commitment to honoring the body
as the temple of the Holy Spirit.

Through my 30-Day program I will teach you
how to live healthier lives by applying biblical principles
to nutrition, exercise, and daily habits. The program is
designed to help believers understand that the foods God
created are meant to heal the body, not harm it and that
food can be our medicine when used in alignment with
His divine design.

INTRODUCTION

Kingdom Body Renewal Health & Wellness 30-day faith-based program is designed to help you renew your mind, rebuild your body, and your spirit. This program is not a diet it's a spiritual transformation journey built upon God's Word.

As believers, we are called to honor God with every part of our lives, including how we care for our physical bodies. Our bodies are sacred vessels, temples of the Holy Spirit. When we learn to live from a place of discipline, balance, and stewardship, we become better equipped to serve the Kingdom.

Kingdom Body Renewal Ministry

✝ ### 30-Day Health & Wellness Transformation Program

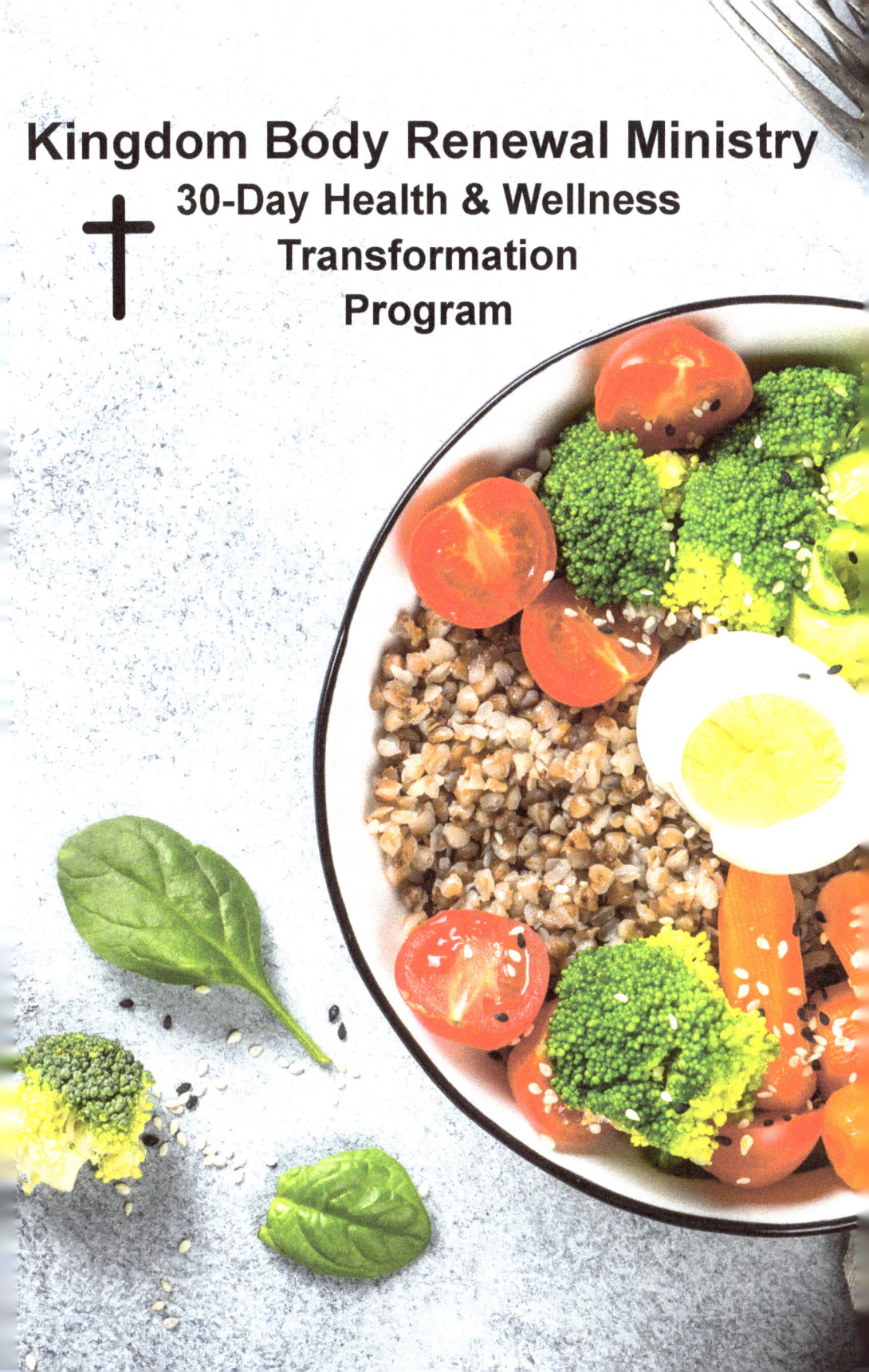

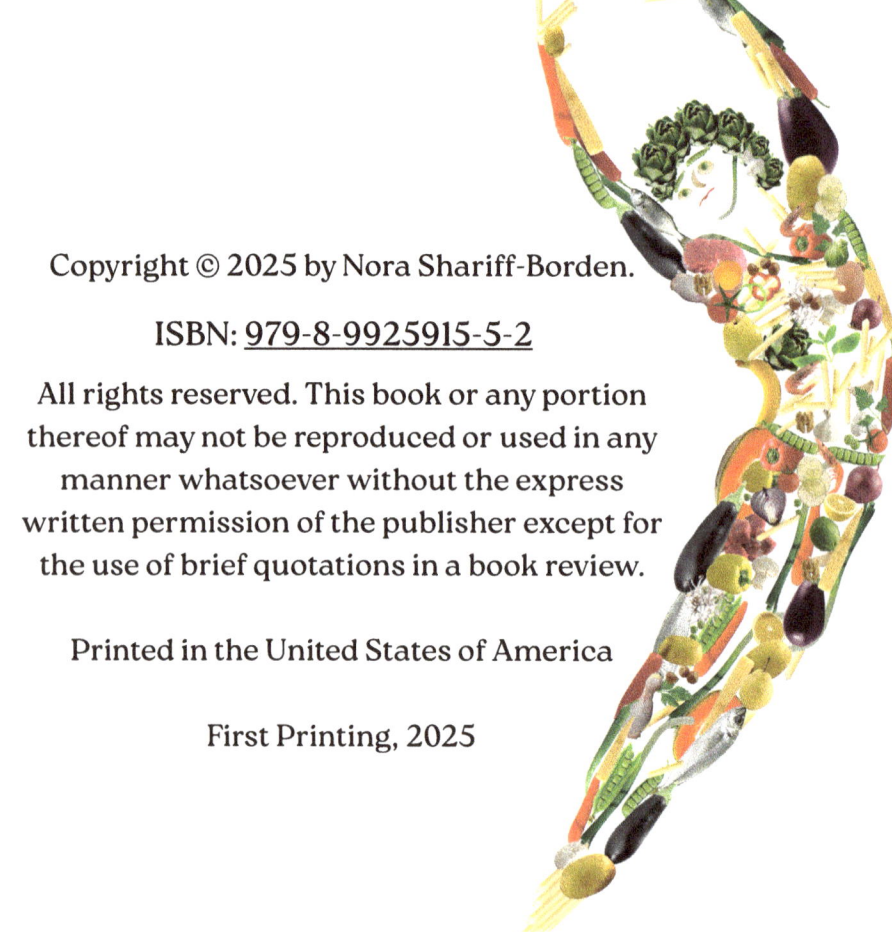

This program will give you the tools to reset your mindset

This program will reset your mindset about food, fitness, water and faith. Develop consistent healthy habits through structure and accountability. It will help you understand how spiritual growth and physical wellness work together. Learn how detoxing your body, fasting, prayer, and nutrition align with God's principles of health. By the end of this journey, your transformation will not only be seen in your body, but felt in your confidence, peace, and purpose.

Key Principle: Transformation is not about perfection it's about progress in partnership with God.

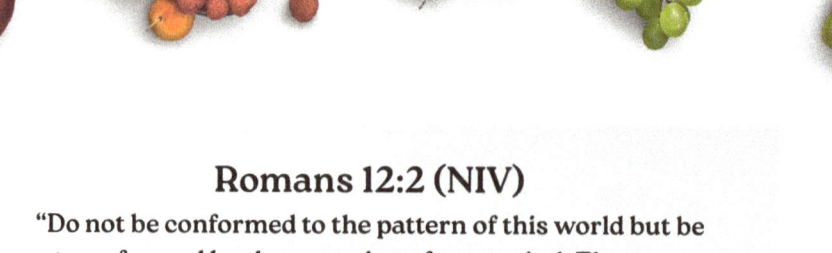

Romans 12:2 (NIV)

"Do not be conformed to the pattern of this world but be transformed by the renewing of your mind. Then you will be able to test and approve what God's will is. His good, pleasing and perfect will."

Transformation begins with what we believe. The world promotes temporary results, but God's plan is a lasting change that starts from within. As you renew your mind through Scripture, you will begin to make decisions that align with His purpose for your health.

1 Corinthians 6:19–20 (NIV)

"Do you not know that your bodies are temples of the Holy Spirit, who is in you, whom you have received from God? You are not your own; you were bought at a price. Therefore, honor God with your bodies."

Your health is a form of worship. Every meal, movement, and moment of self- control is an act of obedience.

3 John 1:2 (AMP)

"Beloved, I pray that in every way you may succeed and prosper and be in good health (physically), just as I know your soul prospers (spiritually)."

This verse reflects God's desire for balance spiritual, emotional, and physical prosperity.

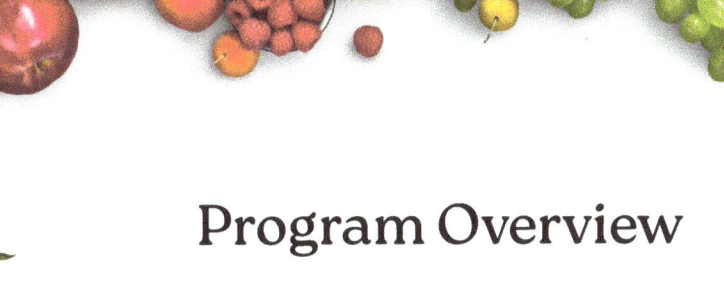

Program Overview

This 30-day program will guide you step-by-step through a process of renewing, honoring, preparing your mind, body and spirit, to walk in wholeness.

Each week includes:

1. A spiritual and physical focus.

2. Practical assignments
 (Detoxing Meal Guidance,
Fasting, and Physical Activity).

3. Reflection questions and
affirmations.

4. A weekly prayer and declaration.
You'll have opportunities to record your
goals, progress, and reflections as you
grow.

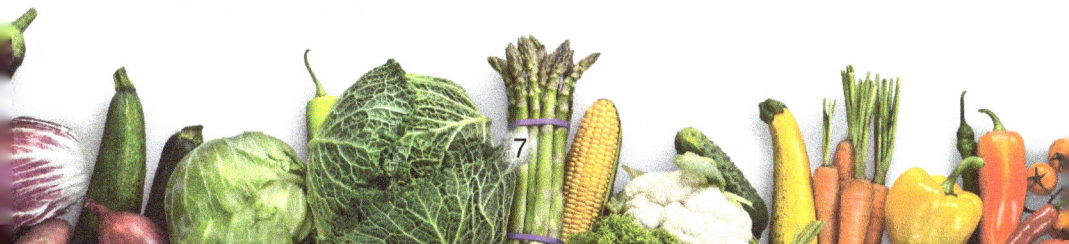

AFFIRMATION #1

SACRED VESSEL AFFIRMATION

My Body Is a Temple of the Holy Spirit, divinely created and uniquely designed by God. I recognize that it is not my own, but a vessel entrusted to me to honor, nurture, and protect. Therefore, I make a conscious and spiritual decision to treat my body with the utmost respect, care, and reverence. I will honor this precious temple by choosing a lifestyle that reflects my gratitude to God for the gift of health and life. My desire is to live a full, vibrant, and balanced life one that glorifies God in both body and spirit. I am committed to eating clean and nourishing foods that fuel my body, restore my energy, and promote healing from within. I understand that what I consume directly impacts not only my physical health but also my spiritual clarity and emotional well-being.

AFFIRMATION #2

HEAL & HYDRATE

Water will be my daily purifier, cleansing my body and renewing my strength. I will move my body with intention and purpose, knowing that every stretch, step, and exercise strengthens the vessel God has given me to carry out His work. My commitment is to stay active, disciplined, and mindful, ensuring that I am physically able to fulfill the assignments and calling that God has placed upon my life.

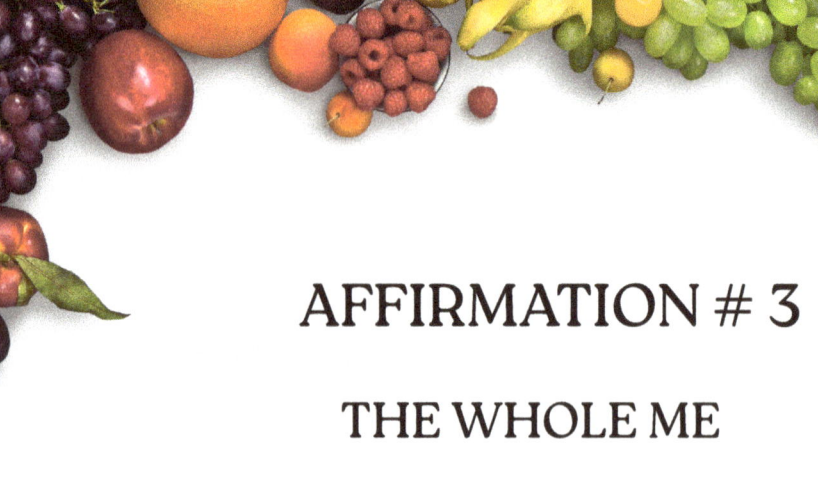

AFFIRMATION # 3

THE WHOLE ME

This journey is not merely about
fitness or appearance, it is
about stewardship. I honor the
Holy Spirit who dwells within
me by living a life that
exemplifies health, self-control,
and obedience. My body, mind,
and spirit will remain aligned
with God's purpose so that I
may continue to walk in divine
health, strength,
and wholeness
all the days of my life.

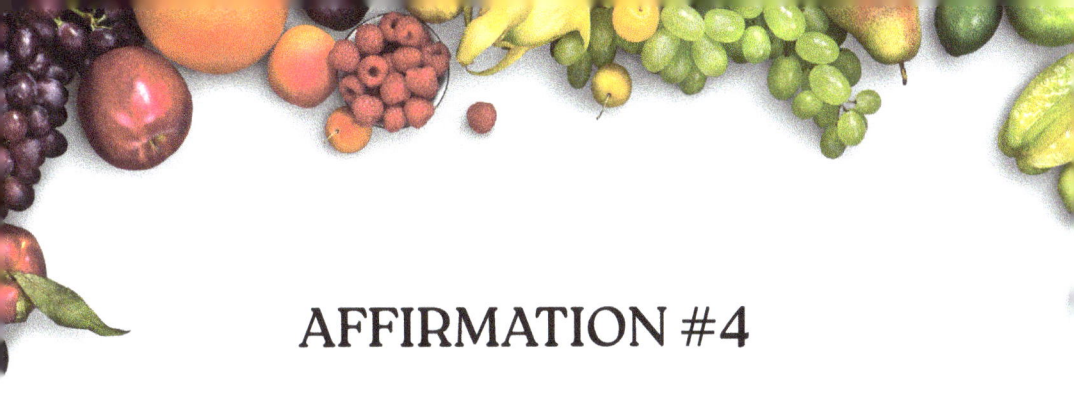

AFFIRMATION #4

DECLARATION

I am grateful for the temple God has given me. I choose to honor it daily through clean eating, hydration, movement, rest, and prayer. I am strong, disciplined, and dedicated to living the abundant, healthy life that God desires for me.

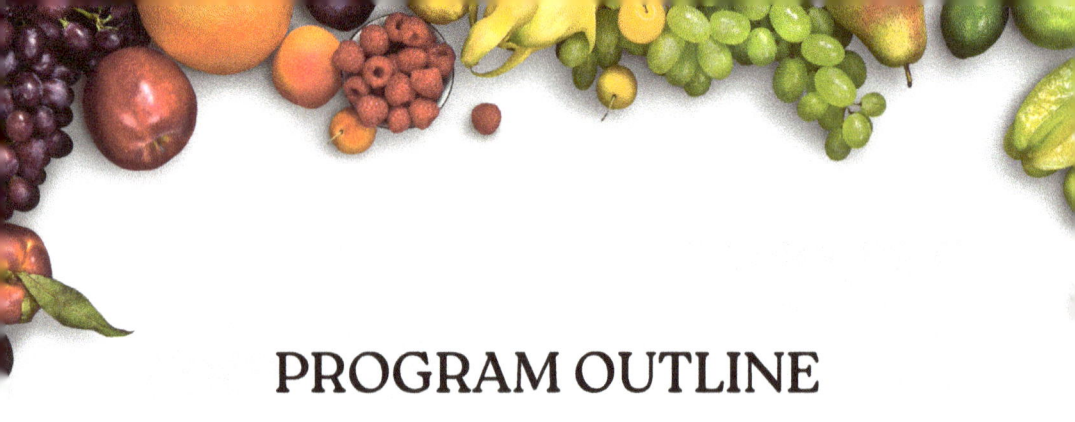

PROGRAM OUTLINE

Week 1 ~ Renewing My Mind

Week 2 ~ Honoring the Temple

Week 3 ~ Prospering in Health

Week 4 ~ Walking in Wholeness

~30 DAY CLOSING PRAYER

~MY REFLECTION & NOTES PAGES

WEEK 1
RENEWING THE MIND

Key Scripture:
Romans 12:2
"Be transformed by the renewing of your mind."
Theme:
How Your Thoughts Shape Your Health an Wellness Journey

How Your Thoughts Shape Your Health & Wellness Journey

Your thoughts have incredible power they shape your emotions, influence your habits, and ultimately determine the direction of your health and wellness
journey. The way you think about yourself, your body, and your abilities can either propel you toward healing and wholeness or hold you back in cycles of doubt and defeat.

How Your Thoughts Shape Your Health and Wellness Journey

Positive, faith-filled thoughts produce
motivation, discipline, and hope. When you
believe that, you can change. You begin to make
better choices like choosing
nourishing foods, staying active, drinking water,
and prioritizing rest. On the other
hand, negative thinking creates stress,
discouragement, and unhealthy habits that
can damage both body and spirit.
The Bible reminds us in
Proverbs 23:7,
"As a man thinketh in his heart, so is he."
This means that your health begins in your
mind. By renewing your thoughts daily
speaking life, declaring health, and aligning your
mindset with God's Word you
position yourself for transformation.
When your thoughts are centered on faith,
gratitude, and discipline, your actions
will follow. Over time, those consistent actions
will build lasting habits that
support a healthy, balanced, and vibrant life
physically, mentally, and spiritually.

How Your thoughts Shape Your Health and Wellness Journey

Renewing the mind means aligning your thoughts with truth. Many people start health programs by focusing on the body, but lasting transformation begins with the mind.

This week's goal is to retrain your thinking about food, discipline, and self-worth. God wants His people to be healthy, strong, and capable of carrying out Kingdom assignments. We cannot do that if we are sick and not healthy.

How Your Thoughts Shape Your Health & Wellness Journey

Renewal happens when you shift your perspective and stop viewing change as punishment but instead see it as God's way of preparing you for something better. Many resist change because it feels uncomfortable or unfamiliar, but true transformation requires a willingness to let go of old habits, mindsets, and routines that no longer serve your health or purpose.

When you begin to see change as preparation, you understand that every step whether it's adjusting your diet, exercising more, or renewing your mind is positioning you for strength, balance, and long-term wellness. God uses the process of change to refine you, discipline you, and teach you how to care for your body as His temple.

This mindset turns frustration into faith and struggle into strength. Renewal is not about loss it's about growth. It's about allowing God to shape you into a healthier, more vibrant version of yourself, ready to live fully and purposefully in the life He has blessed you with.

How Your Thoughts Shape Your Health & Wellness Journey

When your mind is renewed, your choices shift:

• You no longer eat for comfort but for strength.
• You move your body not out of guilt but out of gratitude.
• You learn that every choice brings you closer to or further from your purpose.
• You learn that water is essential part of keeping your temple fully hydrated.
This week is about teaching you about awareness and becoming conscious of your thoughts, words, and habits.

How Your Thoughts Shape Your Health & Wellness Journey

Practical Wellness Assignment

1. Morning Routine:

~Begin each day with prayer and one scripture (Romans 12:2 is your anchor).

~Weigh yourself first thing in the morning this is key it will help keep track of your weight, it will also let know if you need to make any adjustments to what you're eating..

~Drink 8–10 oz. of water before breakfast.

~Also, I would recommend that you drink a hot cup of water with slices lemons or limes.

~Take 3 deep breaths and speak your daily affirmation over your life, goals, and wellness.

2. Nutrition Focus:

~I suggest you start your day with eating fruit.

~Meals should be 80% vegetables fruits and 20% protein.

~Avoid processed foods, sugar, and caffeine.

~Drink half your body weight of water in ounces daily.

3. Detox Focus:

~Select two detox days (I would recommend https://doctorjoesdetox.com)

~Pray during your meal times, asking the Holy Spirit to cleanse your spirit as your body detoxes.

Movement Assignment:

~ Exercise 3-4 times this week (walking, stretching, or cardio).

~ Focus on consistency, not perfection each session is a seed of obedience.

"In Him we live and move and have our being."

Acts 17:28

Set Three Goals for the Week

1.
2.
3.

My Reflection

What habits or thoughts have hindered my growth in the past?

How is God renewing my thinking about food, health, or discipline?

What did I learn about myself this week?

Prayer Focus

"Heavenly Father, renew my mind and cleanse my heart. Help me to think differently, eat wisely, and move faithfully. I surrender every unhealthy pattern and ask You to replace them with purpose, peace, and self-control. In The Name and Through The Power Of Jesus Christ, Amen."

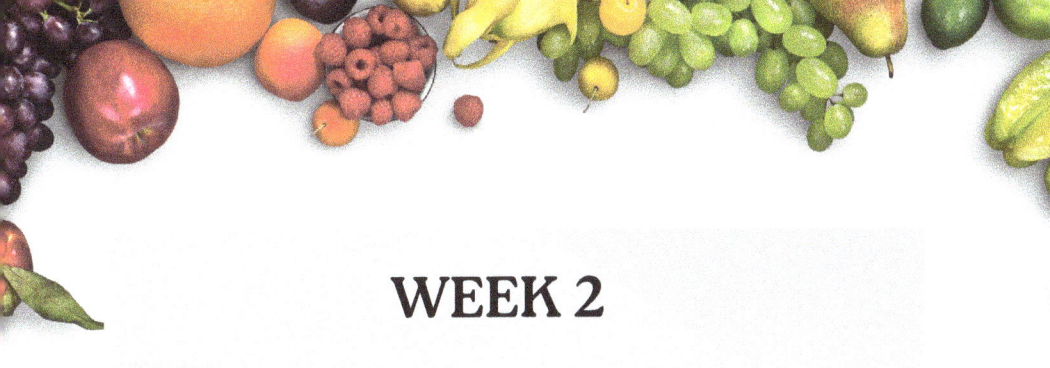

WEEK 2

Honoring the Temple
1 Corinthians 6:19-20

Caring for the Body as a Sacred Vessel

Caring for the body as a sacred vessel begins with understanding that your body is not just flesh and bone it is a divine creation, a home for the Holy Spirit, and a reflection of God's love and craftsmanship. To truly honor your body, you must see it through spiritual eyes, not through the lens flesh, frustration, disappointment, or comparison.

Ask yourself: How do I treat my body when I am disappointed? When I don't like what I see in the mirror? When I've fallen off my goals or failed to see the results I was hoping for? These moments reveal the truth about how you view your body and your relationship with self-care.

For many, disappointment leads to self-criticism, neglect, or giving up altogether. But caring for your body as a sacred vessel means responding with compassion, patience, and grace, especially when you feel discouraged. It means choosing to nourish your body instead of punishing it, to rest instead of overwork, and to speak life instead of words of defeat. When anger or frustration rises because progress feels slow, remember that your body is doing its best to heal, grow, and adapt. Every healthy choice you make every meal prepared with love, every step you take, every moment of stillness and prayer is an act of worship. Your care becomes a daily offering to God, expressing gratitude for the life and strength He has given you.

Treat your body as you would treat something sacred because it is. Be gentle with yourself when you stumble. Offer forgiveness when you fall short. And remind yourself that honoring your body is not about perfection, but about consistent love and stewardship. The goal is not to achieve a certain image but to live in alignment with God's design for health, wholeness, and divine purpose.
Every act of care physical, emotional, and spiritual is a reflection of your understanding that your body truly belongs to Him.
Assignments: 4 meals a day that don't exceed 400 calories each meal don't fall below 200
Exercise 3-4 times a week
"Reflection Question: How do my choices reflect gratitude for my body?"

Prayer: Write a thanksgiving prayer for strength and stewardship.

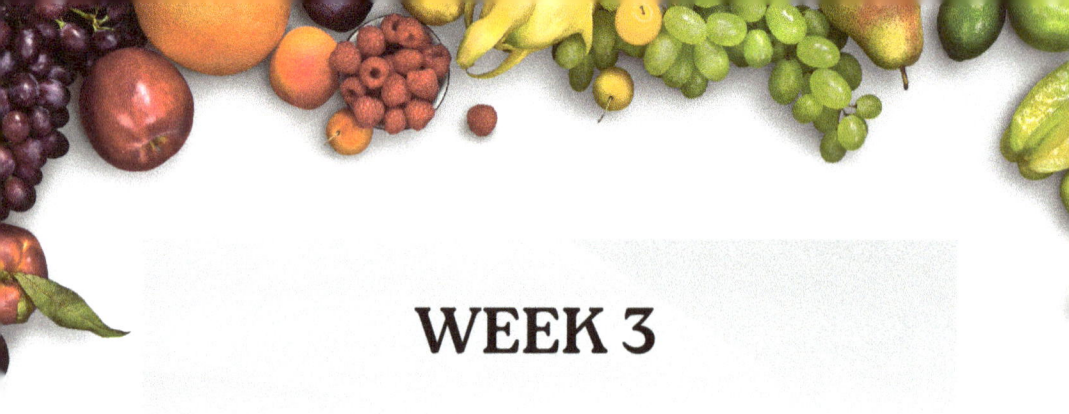

WEEK 3

3 John 1:2

True prosperity in health is not
achieved overnight it blossoms
through daily
consistency and a grateful heart.
These two principles, when
practiced together,
creates a spiritual and physical
harmony that transforms not only
your body but
also your mindset and life.
Consistency builds the foundation
for lasting wellness,
while gratitude keeps your heart
aligned with joy and faith, allowing
abundance
to flow freely into your health
journey.

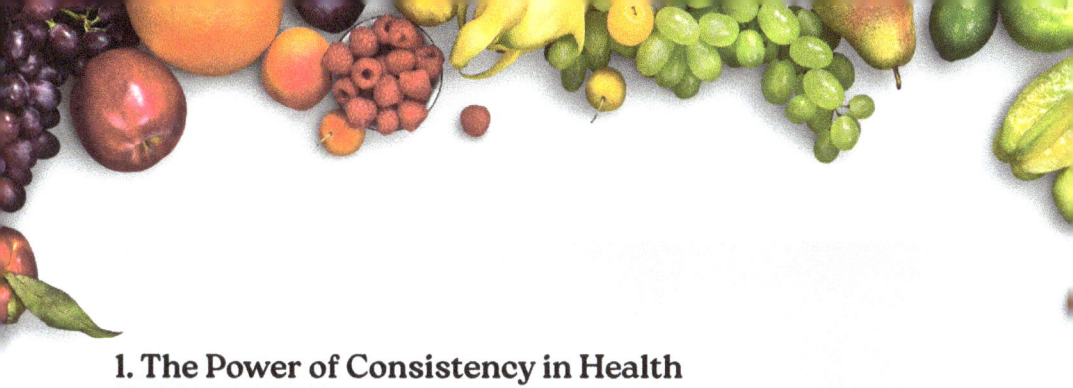

1. The Power of Consistency in Health

Consistency is the bridge between your goals and your results. It's not about perfection, but about persistence making daily decisions that align with your desire for health and wholeness.

~**Physical Consistency:** When you choose to eat nourishing foods, drink water, exercise, and rest, your body begins to trust you. Over time, these choices repair, restore, and strengthen your physical temple.

~**Mental Consistency:** Your thoughts direct your behavior. By maintaining a consistent mindset of discipline, faith, and hope, you silence self-doubt and strengthen your belief that change is possible.
When you consistently honor your body as God's temple, your actions become acts of worship. This spiritual discipline creates alignment between your faith and your lifestyle, drawing divine strength to sustain your journey. Remember, small steps taken consistently lead to big transformations. When you show up every day whether to move your body, prepare a healthy meal, or pray for renewal you build momentum that turns habits into a lifestyle.

Spiritual Consistency

2. The Role of Gratitude in Health:
Gratitude is a powerful spiritual medicine that heals the mind, renews the spirit, and even influences the body's chemistry. Studies show that a thankful heart reduces stress, boosts the immune system, and promotes better sleep but beyond science, gratitude is a key to spiritual prosperity.

~Emotional Healing: Gratitude shifts your focus from what's wrong to what's right. Instead of criticizing your body for what it isn't, you begin to thank God for what it is capable of.

~ Faith Activation: When you express gratitude for small victories like choosing water over soda or walking 10 minutes longer you invite God to multiply your progress.

~Joy and Motivation: Gratitude keeps your heart light. When you wake up thankful, you approach your health journey not as a burden but as a blessing.

A grateful mindset turns everyday actions like preparing meals or exercising into moments of praise, connecting your physical renewal to your spiritual purpose.

3. How Consistency and Gratitude Work Together:

Consistency without gratitude can feel like pressure. Gratitude without consistency can feel like wishful thinking. But together, they create balance and prosperity in health.

~Consistency builds structure; gratitude builds spirit.

~Consistency produces progress; gratitude produces peace.

~Consistency changes your habits; gratitude changes your heart.

When you practice both, your journey becomes sustainable. You stop chasing perfection and start living in divine rhythm where discipline is guided by love, and every act of self-care becomes an offering of worship.

4. The Prosperity That Follows:

Prosperity in health goes beyond the absence of illness it means thriving in every area of life. When you combine consistency and gratitude:

~Your body gains strength and energy.

~Your mind becomes clear and focused.

~Your spirit walks in alignment with God's will for your life.

This prosperity isn't just physical it's emotional, spiritual, and relational. You begin to glow from the inside out, attracting blessings, peace, and favor because you're living with intention and thanksgiving.

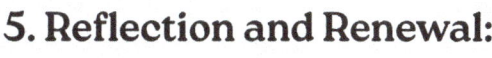

5. Reflection and Renewal:

Ask yourself:

~Am I showing up daily for my health with faith and discipline?

~Do I thank God for the progress I've already made, even if it's small?

~How can I bring more gratitude into my daily health routine?

When you find the balance between being consistent in your actions and grateful in your heart, you'll discover that prosperity was never far away it was waiting for you to align your habits with your faith.

Conclusion:

Finding consistency and gratitude is about more than health it's about stewardship. You are honoring the temple God has given you. Every time you make a healthy choice, speak life over your body, or give thanks for the progress you've made, you are planting seeds of prosperity. Over time, these seeds grow into strength, peace, and radiant health

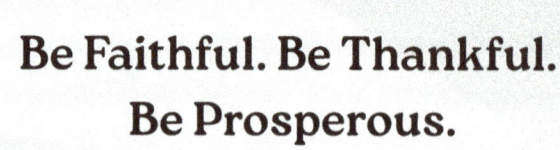

Be Faithful. Be Thankful.
Be Prosperous.

The Importance of Fruit Fasting
One Day per Week.

Taking one day each week to fast on fruit and water is a powerful way to give your body and spirit a much-needed reset. This gentle practice allows your digestive system to rest, your cells to repair, and your mind to refocus on balance and discipline.

1. Physical Renewal:

Fruit fasting provides the body with essential vitamins, minerals, and natural
sugars while allowing digestion to slow down. This rest period helps detoxify the liver, flush out toxins, and improve digestion. Fruits like apples, oranges, grapes, and berries hydrate and cleanse the system, while water assists in removing waste and purifying the bloodstream.

2. Mental and Emotional Clarity:

Taking a break from heavy foods gives the brain a sense of calm and clarity. Many people experience heightened focus, reduced stress, and an overall feeling of lightness. It's a reminder that self-control and simplicity can strengthen your mental and emotional resilience.

3. Spiritual Connection:

Fasting, even for one day, reconnects you with God and helps shift your focus from physical desires to spiritual nourishment. It becomes a time of prayer, gratitude, and reflection—allowing the Holy Spirit to renew your strength from within.

4. Long-Term Benefits:

Over time, this weekly rhythm promotes better digestion, improved energy, clearer skin, and stronger immunity. It teaches consistency, self-discipline, and the importance of honoring your body by giving it rest and renewal.
Taking just one day a week for fruit and water fasting is not deprivation it's a sacred act of care that restores balance to your body, mind, and spirit.

Keep A Gratitude Journal.

1. Strengthens a Positive Mindset:

Keeping a gratitude journal helps you focus on what's going right instead of what's wrong. Writing down daily blessings big or small trains your mind to see God's goodness at work in every situation and builds emotional resilience.

2. Promotes Inner Peace and Joy:

Reflecting on moments of gratitude reduces stress and anxiety. It shifts your thoughts from worry to thankfulness, allowing peace and joy to flow more freely through your heart and mind.

3. Encourages Consistency in Faith and Growth:

A gratitude journal helps you stay consistent in recognizing God's faithfulness.
Over time, it becomes a powerful record of answered prayers and personal growth, reminding you how far you've come and how blessed you truly are.

The Importance Of Sharing Your Testimony With Others:

1. Inspires and Strengthens Others:

Sharing your testimony allows others to see how God has worked in your life. Your story can give someone hope, encouragement, and the faith to believe that if God did it for you, He can do it for them too.

2. Deepens Your Own Faith:

When you speak about what God has brought you through, it reminds you of His power and faithfulness. Testifying renews your gratitude and strengthens your trust in Him for future challenges.

3. Glorifies God and Builds Community:

Your testimony gives glory to God by showing His grace in action. It also helps build connection and unity among believers, creating a community rooted in shared faith, healing, and victory.

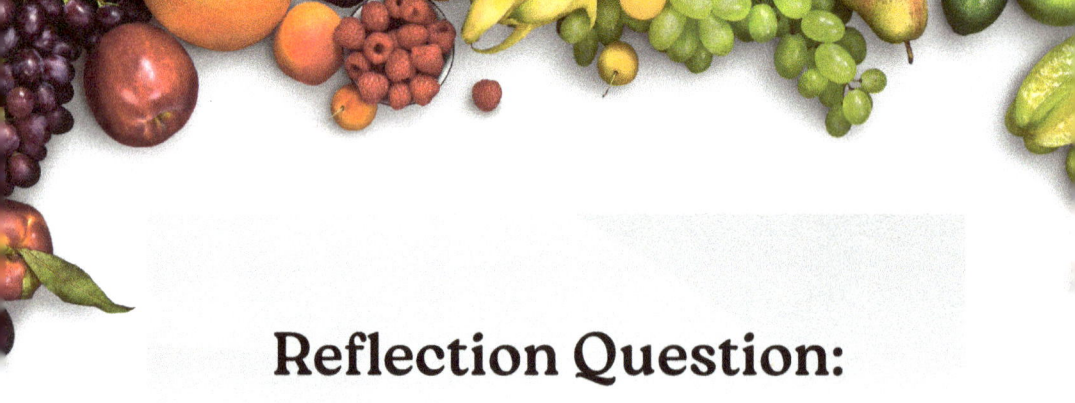

Reflection Question:

**"I Want You To Take 5 Mins and Share
The Changes That You Have Notice
Since Beginning This Journey?"**

Closing Prayer:

Heavenly Father,
Give me the strength to endure every challenge
with grace and faith. When I feel
weary, remind me that Your power is made
perfect in my weakness. Help me find
balance in my mind, body, and spirit so that I
may walk in peace and purpose.
Guide my steps, renew my energy, and let Your
presence keep me centered in all I
do. In Name And Power Of Jesus Christ, Amen.

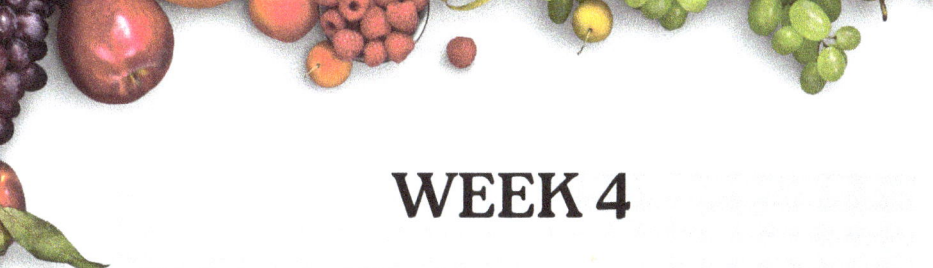

WEEK 4

Walking in Wholeness

Key Scripture: Philippians 1:6
being confident of this, that he who began a good work in you will carry it on to completion until the day of Christ Jesus.

Maintaining Progress on Your New Health Journey Through Grace:

Beginning a health journey is one thing but maintaining it requires something deeper than will power it requires grace. Grace reminds us that transformation is not about perfection but about progression. It teaches us to embrace the process, to be kind to ourselves when we fall short, and to keep moving forward with faith and consistency.

1. Understanding Grace in Your Health Journey

Grace means giving yourself permission to grow at your own pace. It's the divine reminder that God's strength is made perfect in your weakness. When you make a mistake skip a workout, overeat, or lose focus grace whispers, "Start again." Your health journey isn't defined by one bad day but by your willingness to get back up and try again. Grace allows you to shift from guilt to gratitude, from shame to self-compassion, and from pressure to peace.

2. Letting Go of Perfection and Embracing Progress

Too often, people expect overnight results. But health is not a race it's a lifelong relationship with your body, mind, and spirit. Grace helps you celebrate small victories along the way. Every pound lost, every healthy meal, every moment of discipline is a step toward wholeness. Instead of condemning yourself for not being where you want to be, celebrate how far you've come. God is pleased with progress, not perfection.

3. Inviting God into the Process

Maintaining your progress means surrendering your health journey to God daily. Ask Him for strength when you feel weak, discipline when you feel distracted, and peace when you feel overwhelmed. Grace flows when you acknowledge that this journey is not just about your body it's about honoring the temple He created. Prayer, scripture, and reflection keep your focus centered on Him rather than on external results.

4. Extending Grace to Your Body

Your body will change over time sometimes quickly, sometimes slowly. Grace means listening to your body with love instead of criticism. Rest when you need, nourish it with whole foods, and move it with joy. When you operate in grace, you don't punish your body; you partner with it. You realize that healing and growth take time, and that consistency in love will always yield lasting transformation.

5. Renewing Your Mind Daily

Grace renews your mindset by reminding you that your health is an act of worship. Each day is a new opportunity to choose life, healing, and strength.

Romans 12:2 says, "Be transformed by the renewing of your mind."

When you fill your thoughts with positivity, faith, and gratitude, you align your heart with God's plan for your health. Grace helps you see that even when progress is slow, purpose remains.

6. The Gift of Community and Accountability

Grace also works through others. Surround yourself with people who encourage, uplift, and walk with you. Accountability partners or support groups remind you that you're not alone. Sharing your struggles and victories helps you stay grounded in grace rather than isolation or comparison.

7. Grace Brings Balance and Longevity

Without grace, your journey can become a cycle of striving and burnout. With grace, it becomes a lifestyle of balance, peace, and joy. Grace teaches you to rest when needed, eat mindfully, move with intention, and give thanks for every step forward.

Reflection Question:

How can you show yourself more grace this week as you pursue your health goals?

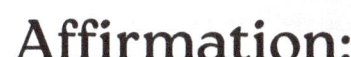

Affirmation:

I am progressing by God's grace. Each day I am
becoming stronger, healthier, and
more aligned with His purpose for my life.

Scripture:

2 Corinthians 12:9
"My grace is sufficient for you, for my power is
made perfect in weakness."

Reflection Question:

"What does wholeness look like for me?"

Closing Prayer:

Lord, help me to keep my body healthy and
strong by eating the foods You created for
me to eat. Remind me that my body is a
temple of Your Spirit. Teach me to honor it
with wisdom, discipline, and gratitude.
Help me to surrender my desires to Your
will and not be ruled by my flesh.
In the name and through the power of the
Holy Spirit,
Amen.

Notes

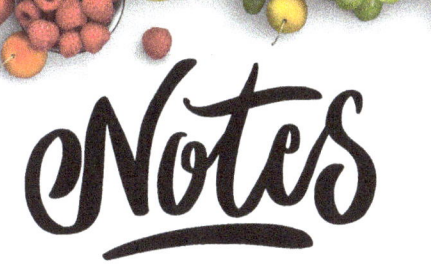

Notes

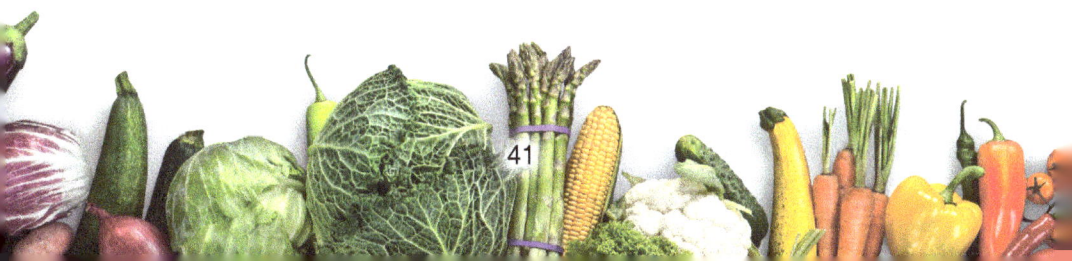

Notes

Notes

Dr. Nora Believes that "Great things happen when people have Great Expectations!"

Stay in touch with Dr. Nora Shariff-Borden and Business Women On The Move For God by following along at:

Instagram @bwotmfg
Facebook @BusinessWomenontheMoveforGod
YouTube @NoraShariff3505
You can also visit https://www.bwotmfg.com/
Spiritualtouchtv.com

Dr. Nora Shariff-Borden
Founder of Kingdom Body Renewal Ministry
Stone Mountain, GA
Info@kingdombodyrenewalministry.com